The Comprehensive Lymphedema and Lipedema Guide

A Simplified Diet Guide with Healthy Recipes for Managing Lymphedema and Lipedema

TABLE OF CONTENTS

Introduction

Lipedema is a complex fat-related disorder that can lead to serious infection if left untreated for an extended time. It is commonly referred to as a fat illness because it is caused by fat accumulation.

Males are more likely to have this condition than females, and minor cases can be treated and controlled with proper nutrition.

Aside from diet, there are food supplements that can help you achieve your ideal physique.

This book provides a comprehensive explanation of Lymphedema and Lipedema, including their causes, symptoms, prevention, therapy, and other useful information for getting back in shape and, most importantly, living a healthy lifestyle.

If you have Lymphedema or Lipedema, it also provides dietary advice, such as what foods to eat and what foods to avoid.

Lymphedema

Lymphedema is a swelling condition caused by an accumulation of protein-rich fluid in the tissues. It is primarily caused by abnormal lymph node tissue production, which reduces lymph fluid flow in the lymphatic system.

It can also affect the legs and arms, as well as the face, mouth, chest wall, neck, trunk, belly, and genitals in some cases. It usually affects one of the arms or legs, though it can affect both arms and legs in some cases. Although it has been reported previously, it only occurs on occasion in the face, chest, neck, genitals, and trunk.

Lymphedema is known to progress in four stages:

Stage 1: This stage starts with abnormal flow or drainage of lymph fluid in the lymphatic system. There are no signs and symptoms in this stage.

Stage 2: Accumulation of lymph fluid, which then leads to swelling due to injury or blockage of the lymph nodes or vessels. The swelling resolves with elevation, and when pressing the affected area a dent might be formed.

Stage 3: The swelling becomes permanent, and it does not resolve with elevation. Dents no longer form when pressing the skin of the affected area, and the skin begins to thicken and scar.

Stage 4: Development of elephantiasis, in which the affected limb is excessively large and malformed, the skin thickens more, and wart-like growth begins to form on the skin leading to excessive scarring.

Lipedema

Lipedema is a condition in which excess fat in the body accumulates in the skin of the lower limbs. During this process, excess body fat migrates from the upper to the lower body. Fat accumulation can be uneven, resulting in unsightly puffiness where fat accumulates. The affected areas include the upper arm, legs, thigh, and buttocks.

Lipedema is most commonly found in the buttocks. After some time, bodily fluid retention is possible in the many swollen areas affected by lipedema.

The main disadvantages of lipedema are discomfort and the fact that it alters a person's normal posture, making it difficult to perform tasks properly. Lipedema is a condition that causes a lot of pain, irritation, and sensitivity in the body. This issue is also responsible for how easily people with this condition bruise. It interferes with their daily tasks, preventing them from being as productive as they could be.

Lipedema is more common in women than in men, with approximately 11% of women suffering from the disease. Lipedema affects the majority of women while they are still young girls, at the beginning of puberty.

This is primarily due to hormonal changes that occur during puberty.

It is critical to distinguish lipedema from obesity or lymphedema. Lymphedema is a condition that causes swelling in the legs to harden without causing pain.

Lipedema can affect people of all sizes and shapes, including the underweight and obese.

This implies that a "normal" weight person could develop lipedema.

Lipedema causes flat feet, knock knees, and joint problems, making it difficult to walk, run, or jog.

Causes of Lymphedema

Some of the most common causes of lymphedema are as follows:

- **Cellulitis** is a common and potentially dangerous bacterial skin infection that causes scarring by causing damage to the tissues surrounding the lymphatic system. Infection with parasitic worms that resemble threads can cause clotting or blockage of lymph nodes and arteries.

- **Cancer cells** growing in the tissues surrounding lymph nodes or veins can clog the lymphatic system and obstruct proper lymph fluid flow.

- **Cancer radiation therapy:** When a cancer tumor is near the lymphatic system, scarring or inflammation of lymph nodes or vessels can occur during the process of using radiation to destroy cancer cells.

- **Inflammatory diseases,** such as Rheumatoid arthritis, are known to cause tissue swelling, which can cause long-term harm to the lymphatic system.

Causes of Lipedema

The causes of lipedema are unknown, and no definitive findings have been made.

Lipedema's causes are similar to those of other illnesses. Lipedema is caused by hormonal changes rather than being overweight.

Even though more than half of lipedema patients are overweight, it is possible to be overweight and healthy. Pregnancy, surgical trauma, and other factors can all contribute to lipedema.

Menopause causes changes in the body's systems as a result of hormonal changes that occur as a result of puberty. Lipedema has no known cause, so the likelihood of developing it varies from person to person and family to family.

Lipedema does not only affect obese people; as previously stated, it can also affect those who appear to be "healthy or normal" in weight. Lipedema is also highly inheritable and heritable, according to research.

Symptoms of Lipedema

The symptoms of lipedema include the following:

- Asymmetry in the upper-to-lower body ratio

- Inability or difficulty in walking,

- Veins that are abnormally enlarged or dilated,

- aches and pains in the swelling areas

- Skin softening and soreness around the afflicted areas

- Sores in the affected areas are uncomfortable.

- Swelling of the damaged areas in a symmetrical pattern,

- The dimpled appearance of the skin on the legs is known as cellulite.

- Touch and feel sensitivity in the afflicted areas

Treatment of lymphedema and Lipedema

Lipedema currently has no treatment options. Everything is being done to treat lipedema and keep it from worsening. There are several things that can be done to lessen the severity of the injury and keep it from getting worse.

Planning your treatment is a collaborative effort, which is why we want you to know that you have options for managing lipedema that will allow you to live a normal, healthy life. The severity of your condition and how it affects your day-to-day life will influence the treatment options available to you. Diet and exercise modifications can be implemented early on to see how your body responds. Fluid-filled areas can also benefit from lymphatic massage. Liposuction is the most effective, first-line treatment for lipedema. If you want to learn more about the diagnosis and treatment of lipedema, please contact your doctor.

Non-Surgical Treatments

Once you have a lipedema diagnosis or are in the diagnostic process, there are nonsurgical treatments you can implement into your daily routine that may soothe some of your symptoms. While nonsurgical methods will not produce the same results as surgery, they can certainly relieve some of the symptoms and pressure associated with this disorder.

1. Exercise

Lipedema patients can benefit from exercises such as swimming, yoga, aqua aerobics, reformer Pilates, and/or walking. It's fine if you prefer a specific type of exercise. You can do whatever exercise suits your needs as long as you feel confident in your ability to perform the movements consistently (even if it is a walk around the block). Building muscle in your legs can also help you fight your lipedema. The key is to keep your mobility intact. Please do not hesitate to ask for more information on what type of exercise is best for lipedema.

2. Diet Changes

Restricting calories may work to take some of the regular fat off your body. Lipedema fat is different. Eating foods with anti-inflammatory properties may help with symptomatic flare-ups and pain. Being mindful of your calorie intake can also assist in the management of your weight. Gaining weight is not ideal.

3. Decongestive massage for the lymphatic system

You (or a trained massage therapist) can manually stimulate drainage, improve blood circulation, and improve lymph fluid flow by manipulating the lymphatic system's trigger points. To encourage more outflow, this intervention works best in the early stages of lipedema and can include dry brushing and whole-body vibration therapy. Later stages of the disease may be too swollen, sensitive to touch, or severe for drainage massage.

4. Medication and Supplement

Lipedema, which is caused by a change in your hormones, can indicate that your hormones are not functioning properly. You may have to run a test on your blood panel to check your hormone levels based on your symptoms. Following this test, some supplements may be recommended to you for boost. Lipedema can take over a healthy immune system due to the influx of inflammation. When you have lipedema, you must take care of yourself. With a weakened immune system, you are more susceptible to infection, slow healing wounds, and illnesses that take longer to recover from.

5. Wearing Compression Garments

Even if you have not had fat removal surgery, wearing compression wraps or garments in areas where lipedema fat exists will help to reduce fluid retention. These massaging compression garments, available in flesh tones or black, take some getting used to, but most are made of a breathable, stretchy fabric that moves with you. You can buy medical compression sleeves that tie at the shoulder or go up the length of your arm to the underarm if you have arm lipedema. Lipedema of the legs can affect the entire length or sections of the leg. There are several types of leggings available to meet your medical needs, including full coverage (upper torso to ankle), abdomen to knees, and knee to ankle open-toe leggings.

Surgical treatments

Excess fat/ flesh can be removed via surgery. Talk to your doctor to get more information about this process

Lymphedema and Lipedema Nutrition

Self-care and therapy for lymphedema and lipedema require proper nutrition. A basic nutrition guide is provided, which includes nutritional alternatives, foods to eat and avoid, eating habits to change, and lymphedema and lipedema recipes.

Food to Eat and Food to avoid

Every illness has both a nutritional cause and an effect on the body. Our eating habits influence almost every aspect of our lives, if not all. This also applies to lipedema and lymphedema. Some foods can improve your mood, while others can make you feel worse.

Appropriate food and eating habits have long been known to aid in the prevention of lipedema worsening. Although these foods will not cure lipedema, they will help to reduce fat deposition in the affected areas.

Food to eat

Let's take a look at some foods that can be included in the diet of a lipedema patient, specifically the Foods to Eat:

1. Proteins

Protein is one of the six nutritional categories, and its role in wound healing, hormone synthesis, and tissue growth is well known. Proteins can only perform specific functions if all of the necessary amino acids are present. A lipedema patient's diet should include a sufficient amount of these essential amino acids to help alleviate symptoms.

For lipedema patients, eggs, particularly egg white, are a good source of protein. Egg whites are high in essential amino acids as well as minerals like vitamin D. Egg whites contain less saturated fat, which is beneficial to those with this condition.

1. Nuts and Seeds:

- Almonds

- Pistachio

- Walnut

- Pecans

2. Proteins:

- egg white

- Beans

- Soy product

- Whole Grains

3. Yogurt

Yogurt is a low-sugar, low-fat food that contains a high concentration of probiotics, which aids in the maintenance of healthy gut microbiota. Only plain and low-fat yogurts are healthy; sweetened yogurts are not.

4. Fruits and vegetables

When it comes to reducing inflammation in the body, fruits and vegetables are one of the best, if not the best, meals to consume. They are rich in antioxidants as well as a variety of micronutrients that support the body's cellular activities.

As long as there are no underlying issues, a lipedema patient can eat any fruit or vegetable, which is correct.

Fruits and vegetables include the following:

- Bell pepper

- Pineapple

- Spinach

- Sweet potatoes

- Tangerine

- Tomatoes

- Orange

- Lemon

- Kale

- Berries

- Any other citrus fruit

5. Whole Grains

Whole grains are grains that have been minimally processed or not processed at all. They still have a lot of fiber, which helps regulate the body's metabolism. Whole grains are an example of this:

- Basmati

- Brown rice

- Oats

- Quinoa

6. Beans

Beans are worth mentioning when it comes to foods that can be consumed. Beans are high in fiber and protein. They can be altered in a variety of ways, resulting in a wide range of consumption options.

Those in the beans family include:

- Black beans

- Chicken peas

- Kidney beans

- Lentils

7. Fish

Oily fish contain omega-3 fatty acids, which are powerful antioxidants and anti-inflammatory agents. Lipedema, a condition caused by the presence of fat in the body, can be treated. These Omega-3 fatty acids help to regulate fat deposition.

Examples of fishes that contain Omega-3 fatty acids are:

- Mackerel

- Anchovies

- Salmon

- Sardines

Food to avoid

Following the topic of foods to include in one's diet, it's critical to understand which foods should be avoided. Among these foods are:

1. Meat

Grain that has been significantly processed or modified has lost most, if not all, of its useful components such as fiber, minerals, and proteins. This can hasten the progression of inflammation in patients while also decreasing the efficacy of other treatments such as compression and exercise.

2. Refined Grains

Refined grains have been heavily processed or altered, causing the majority, if not all, of their beneficial components such as fiber, minerals, and proteins to be lost. This can hasten the progression of inflammation in patients while also decreasing the effectiveness of other treatments like exercise and compression.

3. Dairy Products

Chemicals in dairy meals and products can disrupt or change the gut microbiota. This will accelerate the inflammatory process, causing more discomfort and suffering for a lipedema patient.

As earlier stated, plain yogurt which is a dairy product is exempted from this list due to its beneficial effect.

4. Sugars

This sugar is added to the naturally occurring sugars in the food. Sugar is abundant in some foods, raising blood sugar levels and encouraging the body to store excess fat.

Other foods that should be refrained from include:

- Processed foods

- Excess Salt

Cutting carbs and replacing them with proteins, fruits, and vegetables can help you eat a better diet in addition to all of this.

There are a few things you can do at home to help lessen lipedema symptoms before you look into more intrusive treatments, and every little bit helps! Your diet has a big influence on when and how much your body expands, and the food you eat is a big part of it.

The RAD diet (Rare Adipose Disorder Diet)

A RAD diet is a modified Mediterranean diet that helps keep blood sugar levels stable and prevents blood sugar spikes. To accomplish this, avoid refined or processed carbohydrates and sweets. They can be found in rice, bread, corn, potatoes, and pasta. Avoiding processed foods, particularly processed carbohydrates, will assist you in maintaining a healthy insulin level and reducing pain.

According to lipedema and lymphedema doctors, simply avoiding carbohydrates will not prevent symptoms from worsening. Patients with lipedema and lymphedema should avoid gluten as much as possible. Gluten is most commonly found in wheat, rye, and barley. Replace gluten in your diet with foods high in omega-3 fatty acids and fiber to help your body burn fat and reduce inflammation.

Colorful foods, such as nuts, beans, fish, whole grains, nuts, and seafood, should be prioritized.

Because lipedema primarily affects a woman's lymphatic system, some such foods can be harmful to her health. Just two of the things that can aggravate lipedema symptoms are refined sugar and highly processed foods. While treatment and daily factor options vary from patient to patient, specific dietary programs, such as the RAD diet for lipedema, have proven to be effective for some women. The RAD (Rare Adipose Disorder) diet is designed to reduce inflammation and fluid retention in the body while keeping women at their target body weight.

The RAD diet for lipedema involves avoiding the following foods:

✓ high-fat animal meat (particularly bacon, sausage, and red meat)

✓ Highly processed or salty foods

✓ Lactose-free dairy products (milk, cheese, and yogurt)

✓ Sugars and simple carbohydrates (pasta, white rice, potatoes, honey, or cereals)

✓ Products made from wheat or processed flour (white tortillas or white bread)

Diet Supplements on Lymphedema and Lipedema Diet

Taking a vitamin supplement on a regular and sufficient basis, in addition to the RAD diet, is another tool in your edema-fighting arsenal. These vitamin supplements are inexpensive and can be purchased at your local drugstore.

Vitamin D3 deficiency is common in lipedema patients. **Vitamin D** is an important nutrient that helps your immune system. It is also beneficial to the nervous system, muscles, bones, and muscles. Lipedema patients who are vitamin D deficient should take up to four times the RDA.

Selenium is a mineral that can aid digestion. It has been shown to help people with lipedema reduce swelling, which is usually painful and continuous. While more tablets are tough to come by, brazil nuts contain them; just two of these nuts every day should be enough.

Diosmin: A bioflavonoid found in citrus fruits, diosmin is possibly the most helpful supplement. They have anti-inflammatory, antioxidant, and lymphatic properties, which can help with lipedema symptoms.

Recipes

Roasted Vegetable Crostini

- 1 onion, sliced

- ¾ teaspoon salt

- ½ cup chopped fresh basil

- ¼ teaspoon black pepper

- ¼ cup grated Parmesan cheese

- 1 teaspoon dried oregano

- 1(1-pound) eggplant, diced

- 12 pitted Kalamata olives, halved

- 2 red bell peppers, finely chopped

- 8 ounces Italian bread, cut into 24 thin slices and toasted

- 2zucchini, finely chopped

- 2 tablespoons extra-virgin olive oil

Direction

1. Preheat the oven to 425°F.

2. Combine the onion, zucchini, eggplant, bell peppers, oil, black pepper, oregano, and salt in a large roasting pan. Spread out to form a single layer. Vegetables should be roasted for 45 minutes, stirring occasionally, until soft and browned on the edges. Allow to come up to room temperature.

3. Distribute the vegetable mixture evenly on the toast. Olives, basil, and Parmesan should be evenly distributed.

Lemon-Thyme Zucchini on Flatbread

- 1½ teaspoons extra-virgin olive oil

- ½ teaspoon salt

- ½ teaspoon dried

- ½ cup crumbled soft goat cheese, at room temperature

- 3 tablespoons lemon juice

- 3 garlic cloves, minced

- 2zucchini, cut crosswise

- 2 teaspoons chopped fresh thyme or

- 3whole wheat naan flatbreads

Direction

1. Combine the zucchini, oil, garlic, thyme, salt, and
    lemon juice in a large zip-top plastic bag. Inflate the
    bag, seal it, and then turn it to coat the zucchini. Take
    a 30-minute break.

2. Spray the grill rack with nonstick cooking spray.
    Grills can be preheated to medium-high temperatures,
    or medium-high fires can be prepared directly on the
    grill.

3. Grill the zucchini for 2 minutes per side, or until soft.
    Serve on a platter. Place the naan on the grill rack for
    two minutes, or until the bottom is lightly crisped.
    Turn the naan over and evenly distribute the zucchini
    and goat cheese. Cook the naan for 3 minutes more,

covered until the bottoms are lightly browned.

Crosswise cut the naan in half.

California Sushi Rolls

- ½ cup seasoned rice vinegar

- ½ cucumber, peeled and cut into thick matchsticks

- ½ avocado, peeled, pitted, and cut into thick matchsticks

- ¼ pound surimi (imitation crab), cut into thick matchsticks

- 1 teaspoon Asian (dark) sesame oil

- 1 teaspoon grated peeled fresh ginger 4 (7 × 8-inch) nori sheets

- 2¼ cups water

- 2 teaspoons of wasabi powder

- 2 cups sushi rice, rinsed and drained

- 1tablespoon sesame seeds, toasted

- 2tablespoons reduced-sodium soy sauce

- 3 tablespoons warm water

Direction

1. In a medium saucepan, bring rice and water to a boil. Reduce the heat to low, cover, and cook for 20 minutes, or until the rice is soft and the liquid has been absorbed. Put the rice in a large mixing bowl. Combine the vinegar and sesame seeds in a mixing bowl. Allow the rice mixture to come to room temperature.

2. In the meantime, make the dipping sauce by combining warm water, ginger, wasabi, soy sauce, and sesame oil in a serving bowl.

3. Place 1 nori sheet on a sushi rolling mat with the glossy side facing you and the long side facing you to make sushi rolls. With damp hands, spread 1 cup of spiced rice over the nori, leaving a 1-inch border along the longest side closest to you. 3. Cut a 14-inch slit down the length of the rice and insert a quarter of the avocado, cucumber, and surimi.

4. Roll the mat away from you, keeping the filling in place with your fingers, until the nori ends overlap and form a tight cylinder. Equal, moderate pressure is required to remove the sushi roll from the mat. Using a very sharp knife, cut the sushi into six pieces, moistening it between each cut. Repeat with the remaining nori, cucumber, rice, avocado, and surimi

to make a total of 24 pieces of sushi. Please serve

with dipping sauce.

Herbed wild mushroom oatmeal

- 1 teaspoon fresh rosemary

- 1 teaspoon sea salt

- 3/4 teaspoon ground black pepper

- 3 stalk scallions

- 2 cups Dry Oats

- 12 oz sliced mushrooms

- 4 eggs

- 4 cups water

- 2 teaspoon extra-virgin olive oil

- 2 teaspoon 100% Lemon Juice

Direction

1. In a large saucepan over medium-high heat, heat the oil. Cook until the mushrooms are barely cooked through, about 5 minutes, with the white half of the scallions, lemon juice, and pepper.

2. In a nonstick skillet coated with cooking spray, scramble the eggs while the mushrooms cook.

3. Bring the water, rosemary, and salt to a boil over high heat. Reduce the heat to low and stir in the oats and scallions. Cook for 6 minutes, stirring occasionally, or until the oats are tender.

4. Top each dish with a sprinkle of cheese or an egg. Top with more scallions if desired.

Lentil and Swiss Chard Soup

- ¼ teaspoon salt

- 1 cup dried brown lentils, picked over, rinsed, and drained

- 1 garlic clove, minced

- 1/8 teaspoon black pepper

- 2 cups lightly packed thinly sliced Swiss chard leaves

- 2 teaspoons lemon juice

- 2 teaspoons olive oil 1 onion, chopped

- 4 cups reduced-sodium vegetable broth

Direction

1. Heat the oil in a large saucepan over medium heat. Stir in the onion and garlic for about 5 minutes, or until the onion softens. Bring the lentils and broth to a boil. Reduce the heat to low and cook the lentils for 45 minutes with the lid on.

2. Add the chard, salt, and pepper to the soup and cook for 5 minutes, stirring occasionally, or until the chard is wilted. Stir in the lemon juice.

Quick Gumbo

- ½ cup long-grain white rice

- ½ pound large shrimp, peeled and deveined

- ½ teaspoon dried thyme

- 1 bay leaf

- 2 teaspoons olive oil

- 1 (¼-pound) piece reduced-fat kielbasa, cut into 8 slices

- 1 (14½-ounce) can of crushed tomatoes

- 1 garlic clove, minced

- 1 green bell pepper, chopped

- 1 cup sliced fresh or thawed frozen okra

- 1 celery stalk, chopped

- ¹ 8 teaspoon cayenne

- 1 (5-ounce) skinless boneless chicken breast,

- 2cups reduced-sodium chicken broth

- 6 scallions, sliced

- cut into ½-inch pieces

Direction

1. Over medium heat, heat a large saucepan with oil. Stir in the scallions, garlic, bell pepper, and celery for 5 minutes, or until softened.

2. Bring the broth, okra, thyme, tomatoes, bay leaf, and cayenne pepper to a boil while stirring. Cook for 20 minutes, covered, on low heat.

3. Boil the rice in the broth for 15 minutes with the lid on. Mix in the shrimp, kielbasa, and chicken. Cook, covered, for 5 minutes, or until the shrimp are barely opaque in the center, the chicken is cooked through, and the rice is fluffy. Take out the bay leaf.

Smoky Manhattan-Style Clam Chowder

- 1 carrot, diced

- ⅛ teaspoons black pepper

- 1 (6½-ounce) can of chopped clams

- 1 (½-pound) all-purpose potato, peeled and cut into ½-inch dice

- ½ teaspoon dried oregano

- ½ cup water

- 1 celery stalk, diced

- 1 large garlic clove, minced

- 1 onion, chopped

- 1 small zucchini, diced

- 1(14½-ounce) can of fire-roasted diced tomatoes

- 2 teaspoons olive oil

- 2(8-ounce) bottles of clam juice

Direction

1. Warm the oil in a large saucepan over medium heat. Cook for about 5 minutes, stirring occasionally, after adding the onion and garlic. Cook for about 5 minutes, stirring frequently, until the carrot, potato, zucchini, and celery are tender.

2. After adding the water, oregano, pepper, and tomatoes with juice, bring to a boil. 15 minutes simmering on low heat with a partial cover

3. Clams and their juice should be added now. Cook for 2 minutes, or until thoroughly heated.

Classic Pot Roast

- 1 (14½-ounce) can petite diced tomatoes, drained, juice reserved

- ½ teaspoon dried rosemary

- ½ cup dry red wine

- ¼ teaspoon black pepper

- 1 carrot, chopped

- 1 celery stalk, chopped

- 2 garlic cloves, minced 1 teaspoon dried thyme

- 1 cup reduced-sodium beef broth

- 1 teaspoon salt

- 1(2-pound) bottom or top round beef roast, trimmed

- 2onions, chopped

- 4 teaspoons olive oil

- 6 juniper berries, crushed (optional)

Direction

1. Heat the oil in a Dutch oven over medium heat. Add
    the steak and brown it on all sides for about 6
    minutes before plating. Add the rosemary, celery,
    onions, carrots, garlic, thyme, and juniper, if using,
    after the vegetables have softened, about 10 minutes.
    Cook while stirring constantly.

2. Preheat the oven to medium-high. Add the wine by
    scraping any browned bits from the pot's bottom.
    Return the beef to the saucepan with the remaining
    ingredients and just enough of the leftover tomato
    liquid to cover. Reduce the heat to low, cover, and
    cook for about two hours, or until the meat is tender
    to the fork.

3. Place the meat on a cutting board and cut it into 16 thin slices across the grain. Remove the fat from the gravy. Slowly reheat the beef in the pot over low heat.

Peppered Roast Tenderloin

- 1 tablespoon cracked black peppercorns

- 1 (2½-pound) beef tenderloin, trimmed and tied

- ½ teaspoon salt

- 2 teaspoons finely chopped fresh sage

- 2 teaspoons finely chopped fresh rosemary

- 2 garlic cloves thinly sliced lengthwise

- 2 teaspoons finely chopped fresh thyme

- 4 teaspoons olive oil

Direction

1. Preheat the oven to 425°F.

2. Using a small knife, make tiny slits all over the
    tenderloin; insert a slice of garlic into each slit. all
    over the meat with oil Rub the tenderloin with a
    peppercorn, salt, rosemary, thyme, and sage mixture.

3. In a roasting pan, roast the tenderloin for 10 minutes.
    350°F is an ideal oven temperature. Cook for another
    20 minutes, or until an instant-read thermometer
    inserted into the tenderloin registers 145°F for
    medium. Place on a cutting board for 15 minutes. Cut
    into 20 pieces.

Grilled T-Bone Steak

- 2 teaspoons finely chopped fresh rosemary

- 1 teaspoon olive oil

- 1 (1¼-pound) rib steak, about 1 inch thick, trimmed

- ½ teaspoon salt

- ¼ teaspoon black pepper

- 2 teaspoons finely chopped fresh sage

Direction

1. Nonstick splatter the grill rack Preheat the grill to medium-high or start a direct medium-high fire.

2. To make the rub, combine all of the ingredients, except the meat, in a cup. Rub both sides of the steak. Cook the steak for 5 minutes per side, or until an instant-read thermometer inserted into the center of the steak reads 145°F for medium. Place the steak on a cutting board and set it aside for 5 minutes. Make four equal pieces.

Teriyaki-Flavored Grilled Sirloin

- 1 tablespoon grated peeled fresh ginger

- 1 garlic clove, minced

- 1 (1-pound) boneless sirloin steak, about

- ½ inch thick, trimmed

- 2 tablespoons rice wine vinegar

- $1/3$ cup reduced-sodium soy sauce

- ¼ teaspoon red pepper flakes

- 3 tablespoons dark brown sugar

Direction

1. Spray the grill rack with nonstick cooking spray. Grills can be preheated to medium-high temperatures, or medium-high fires can be prepared directly on the grill. Preheat a nonstick grill pan over high heat as an alternative.

2. To make the marinade, combine the vinegar, soy sauce, garlic, brown sugar, ginger, and pepper flakes in a small saucepan over medium heat. Cook for 5 minutes at low heat. Remove from the heat and set aside to cool completely.

3. Place the steak in a large zip-top plastic bag with the cooled marinade. Seal the bag after turning it to coat the steak. Refrigerate for at least 30 minutes and up to 4 hours, flipping the bag occasionally.

4. Remove the steak from the bag and discard the marinade. Cook the steak for about 5 minutes per side on the grill rack or in the grill pan, or until an instant-read thermometer inserted into the side of the steak reads 145°F for medium. Place the steak on a cutting board and set it aside for 5 minutes. Cut into 12 slices perpendicular to the grain.

London Broil

- 1 (1-pound) top round or sirloin tip steak, trimmed

- ½ teaspoon salt

- ½ cup dry red wine

- ¼ teaspoon black pepper

- 1 garlic clove, minced

- 1 tablespoon chopped fresh rosemary

Direction

1. Place the rosemary, wine, garlic, salt, and pepper in a large zip-top plastic bag. Incorporate the steak. Seal the bag after turning it to coat the steak. Refrigerate for at least 6 hours or up to a day, flipping the bag occasionally.

2. Prepare the broiler.

3. Remove the meat from the bag and discard the marinade. Broil the steak 5 inches from the heat for 4 minutes per side, or until an instant-read thermometer inserted into the center of the steak registers 145°F for medium. Place on a cutting board and set aside for 5 minutes. Make 16 slices with a crosscut.

Conclusion

Lipedema is characterized by bilateral subcutaneous fat depositions in the limbs, as well as pain, sensitivity, and bruising. Even though the disease is still poorly understood, it is frequently overlooked.

Lipedema and lymphedema are fat-related infections that can be managed by limiting fat consumption.

I believe you now have a thorough understanding of lipedema and lymphedema, as well as how to prevent and treat them.

If you have any mild symptoms, consult your doctor and stick to your diet.

www.ingramcontent.com/pod-product-compliance
Lightning Source LLC
Chambersburg PA
CBHW072036150726
47999CB00002B/942